Slow Co _ _ _ _ _

Low Carb Slow Cooker Pork Recipes Full Of Quick &
Easy Cooking Recipes

*(Simple And Delicious Crock-pot Dinner Recipes For
Busy People)*

Lance Jacobs

Table Of Contents

Lemon Scones

Ingredients:

- 2 teaspoon baking powder
- 2 fresh egg, beaten
- 4 tablespoons Swerve
- 2 cups almond flour
- 1 cup of coconut oil
- 2 tablespoons lemon juice
- 2 teaspoon cinnamon powder

Directions:

1. In the mixing bowl, combine the flour with the coconut oil and the other ingredients and stir well.
2. Line the slow cooker with baking paper.
3. Make the ball from the dough and place it in the slow cooker.

4. Cut the dough into 6 scones and close the lid.

5. Cook the scones for 4 hours on High.

6. Then chill the cooked dessert well and cut the dough into scones again.

Nutmeg Raspberry Crisp

Ingredients:

- 1/2 teaspoon of nutmeg ground
- 2 tablespoon of sugar-free maple
- 2 teaspoons of cinnamon ground
- 1/2 teaspoon of ginger ground

syrup

- 1/2 cup of almond flour
- 1/2 cup of brown swerve
- 1/2 cup of unsalted butter, melted
- Pinch of salt
- 1 cup of water
- ¾ cup of walnut meal

Directions:

1. Start by tossing all the Ingredients: together in a suitable bowl.
2. Mix both the mixtures together in a bowl until smooth.
3. Now spread the mixture in a grease Crockpot.
4. Cover its lid and cook for 4 hours on Low setting.
5. Once done, remove its lid of the crockpot carefully.
6. Serve.

Keto Chip Cookies

Ingredients:
- 2 fresh egg, beaten
- 2 tablespoons sugar-free chocolate chips
- 2 teaspoon vanilla extract
- 2 cup almond flour
- 4 tablespoons butter, melted
- 2 tablespoons Erythritol

Directions:

1. Mix the beaten egg and butter.
2. Add the vanilla extract and almond flour.
3. Stir the mixture well and add Erythritol.
4. Mix well and add chocolate chips.
5. Knead the dough and divide into small cookies.

6.   Place the cookies in the slow cooker and cook for 4 hours on High.

7.   Let the cooked cookies cool slightly.

8.   Enjoy!

Keto Almond Scones

Ingredients:
- 2 eggs, beaten
- 2 teaspoon vanilla extract
- 4 tablespoons coconut flour
- 2 oz almonds, chopped
- 1 teaspoon baking soda
- 1 cup almond flour
- 1/2 cup coconut milk

Directions:

1. Combine the baking soda and almond flour.
2. Add the coconut milk and beaten eggs,
3. Add the vanilla extract and stir the mixture gently.
4. Add the coconut flour and almonds.

5.   Stir the mixture and knead into a dough.

6.   Make into small scones and put them in the slow cooker.

7.   Cook the scones for 4 hours on High.

8.   Chill the cooked scones and then remove them from the slow cooker to col slightly.

9.   Enjoy!

Chocolate Crème Brule

Ingredients:

- 1 tablespoon of cocoa powder
- 1 cup of swerve
- 1 tablespoon of grated sugar-free chocolate
- 6 egg yolks
- 2 cups of heavy cream
- 2 tablespoon of vanilla extract

Directions:

1. Start by thoroughly blending all the Ingredients: in a blender until smooth.
2. Now divide the batter into 4 ramekins and place them in the Crockpot.

3.   Cover its lid and cook for 2 hours on Low setting.

4.   Once done, remove its lid of the crockpot carefully.

5.   Allow it to cool and refrigerate for 2 hour.

6.   Serve.

Mini Pumpkin Cakes

Ingredients:

- 1/2 teaspoon ground cardamom
- 2 teaspoon vanilla extract
- ¾ cup almond milk, unsweetened
- 2 tablespoon butter
- 2 oz walnuts, chopped
- 2 oz pumpkin puree
- 6 tablespoons almond flour
- 1 teaspoon baking soda
- 2 teaspoon ground cinnamon

Directions:

1.   Combine the pumpkin puree, almond flour, and baking soda.
2.   Add the ground cinnamon, ground cardamom, and vanilla extract.
3.   Stir the mixture gently and add almond milk and butter.
4.   Add the chopped walnuts and stir the batter until smooth.
5.   Place the mixture into small cake molds and transfer them to a slow cooker.
6.   Cook the cakes for 6 hours on Low.
7.   Cool the cakes slightly and serve!

Gingerbread Cookies

Ingredients:

- 2 cup almond flour
- 4 tablespoons butter
- 2 fresh egg, whisked
- 2 teaspoon baking powder
- 2 teaspoon ground ginger
- 2 teaspoon ground cinnamon
- 2 teaspoon vanilla extract

Directions:

1. Add the ground ginger, ground cinnamon, vanilla extract, almond flour, and baking powder into a large bowl.
2. Stir and add the butter and whisked the egg.
3. Knead into a soft dough.
4. Roll it out with a rolling pin and make the cookies.

5.   Place the cookies in the slow cooker and cook them for 4 hours on High.

6.   Chill the cookies and serve!

Avocado Mousse

Ingredients:

- 4 egg yolks
- 2 tablespoons monk fruit
- 1/2 cup organic almond milk
- 2 avocados, peeled, pitted and mashed
- 1/2 cup heavy cream
- 1 teaspoon almond extract

Directions:

1. In the crockpot, mix the avocados with the cream and the other ingredients, whisk and close the lid.
2. Cook the mixture for 2 hours in Low.
3. Divide into cups and serve cold.

Sesame Cookies

Ingredients:

- 1 teaspoon baking powder
- 2 egg
- 2 teaspoon vanilla extract
- 2 tablespoons coconut flour
- 2 tablespoon butter
- 2 tablespoon sesame seeds

Directions:

1. Mix the coconut flour and butter.
2. Add the baking soda and vanilla extract.
3. Beat the fresh eggs into the mixture.
4. Add the sesame seeds and knead the dough.
5. Roll out the dough and cut out cookies with a cookie cutter.

6.   Place the cookies in the slow cooker and cook them for 2 hours on High.

7.   Chill the cookies and serve!

Pumpkin Cake

Ingredients:

- 6 tablespoons of swerve
- 1 medium banana mashed
- 2 tablespoon of canola oil
- 1/2 cup of Greek yogurt
- 1/2 (30 oz.) can pumpkin puree
- 1 egg
- 1/2 teaspoon of pure vanilla extract

- 1/2 cup of sugar-free chocolate
- 6 tablespoons of unbleached almond flour
- 1/2 teaspoon of salt
- 1 teaspoon of baking soda
- 1/2 teaspoon of baking powder
- 1/2 teaspoon of pumpkin pie spice
- chips

Directions:

1. Separately blend the wet and dry Ingredients: in the mixer.
2. Mix both the mixtures together in a bowl until smooth.
3. Now spread the cake batter in a greased ramekin and place it in the Crockpot.
4. Cover its lid and cook for 4 hours on Low setting.
5. Once done, remove its lid of the crockpot carefully.

6.   Allow it to cool and refrigerate for 2 hour.
7.   Serve.

Low Carb Sweet Pecans

Ingredients:

- ⅛ teaspoon of salt
- 2 egg white
- 2 teaspoons of vanilla
- ⅛ cup of water
- 2 cup of swerve
- 2 cup of brown swerve
- 4 tablespoons of cinnamon ground

Directions:
1.   Start putting all the Ingredients: into the Crockpot.
2.   Cover its lid and cook for 4 hours on Low setting with occasional stirring

3.   Once done, remove the pot's lid and give it a stir.
4.   Serve fresh.

Cocoa Cake

Ingredients:

- 4 tablespoons butter
- 2 eggs, beaten
- 1/2 cup of water
- 2 teaspoon almond extract
- Cooking spray
- 1/2 cup stevia
- 1/2 cup coconut flour
- 2 1 tablespoon cocoa powder
- ¾ teaspoon salt
- 1/2 teaspoon baking soda
- 1 teaspoon lime juice

Directions:

1.   In a bowl mix the stevia with the flour, cocoa and the other ingredients except the cooking spray and blend the mixture with the help of the hand mixer.

2.   Spray the slow cooker bottom with the cooking spray.

3.   Pour the cake mixture in the slow cooker and flatten it with the help of the spatula.

4.   Close the lid and cook the dessert for 5 hours on Low.

5.   Chill the cake well before serving.

Red Berry Gummies

Ingredients:

- 2 teaspoon red food coloring
- 2 tablespoons blueberries puree
- 2 tablespoon stevia
- 2 tablespoon gelatin
- 2 cup of water

Directions:

1. Mix up together the gelatin and 6 tablespoons of water.
2. Stir the mixture and leave it for 25 minutes.
3. Meanwhile, pour the remaining water in the crockpot.
4. Add stevia, berries puree and food coloring.
5. Stir the liquid and cook it for 2 hour on High.

6.   Then switch off the crockpot and add gelatin mixture.

7.   Stir it well until homogenous.

8.   Pour the liquid in the gummy bear's molds and chill until solid.

9.   Discard the gummy bears from the molds and store them in the cool place.

Keto Brownies

Ingredients:

- 2 teaspoon vanilla extract
- 2 teaspoon ground cinnamon
- 2 cup almond flour
- 4 tablespoons butter, melted
- 2 fresh egg, beaten
- 2 tablespoon full-fat cream
- 2 teaspoon baking soda
- 2 oz dark chocolate
- 2 teaspoons liquid stevia

Directions:

1.   Melt the chocolate and mix it with the liquid stevia vanilla extract and ground cinnamon.
2.   Add the butter and almond flour.
3.   Add the egg and cream.
4.   Stir the mixture until smooth.

5.   Transfer the mixture to the slow cooker.

6.   Flatten it gently and cook for 4 hours on High.

7.   Cut the cooked dessert into the servings.

Tender Lime Cake

Ingredients:

- 2 1 cup coconut flour
- 2 teaspoon vanilla extract
- 2 teaspoon baking powder
- 4 tablespoons Erythritol
- 2 lime, sliced
- 2 cup almond milk, unsweetened

Directions:

1.   Combine the almond milk, coconut flour, vanilla extract, baking powder, and Erythritol.
2.   Add the vanilla extract and stir until smooth.
3.   Place the mixture in the slow cooker.
4.   Then place the sliced lime over the cake.

5.   Cook for 4 hours on High.

6.   Check if the cake is cooked and chill.

7.   Slice the cake into servings and enjoy!

Kombucha Cake

Ingredients:

- 1/2 teaspoon baking powder
- 4 eggs, beaten
- 2 tablespoons kombucha
- ¾ teaspoon salt
- 2 cup almond flour
- 1/2 cup coconut flour
- 2 tablespoons Erythritol

Directions:

1.   Mix the almond flour and coconut flour.

2.   Add the Erythritol and baking powder.

3.   Add the kombucha and salt and stir the mixture.

4.   Add the beaten fresh eggs and stir the batter until smooth.

5.   Place the batter in the slow cooker and cook for 4 hours on High.

6.   Chill the cooked cake slightly.

7.   Enjoy!

Cherry Cheese Cake

Ingredients:

- 2 tablespoon of vanilla extract
- 2 cups of mixed nuts, crushed
- 2 tablespoons of unsalted butter, melted
- 2 tablespoons of erythritol
- 1/2 cup of fresh cherries pitted
- 8oz. ricotta cheese
- 1/2 cup of erythritol
- 2 fresh eggs
- 1/2 cup of sour cream

Directions:

1.   Start by blending the Nuts with butter in the mixer.
2.   Spread this Nuts mixture in the greased Crockpot firmly.

3. Now beat the remaining filling Ingredients: except cherries in a blender until smooth.

4. Add this cream filling to the Nutty crust and spread evenly.

5. Cover its lid and cook for 6 hours on Low setting.

6. Once done, remove its lid of the crockpot carefully.

7. Allow it to cool and refrigerate for 2 hour.

8. Garnish with cherries.

Traditional Egg Custard

Ingredients:

- 1/2 teaspoon of cinnamon, ground
- Nutmeg, grated
- Fresh fruits, diced
- 6 fresh eggs
- 1/3 cup of erythritol
- 2 teaspoon of vanilla extract
- 2 pinch salt

Directions:

1. Start by blending all the Ingredients: together in a mixer.
2. Pour this mixture into 4 ramekins and place them in the Crockpot.
3. Cover its lid and cook for 2-4 hours on Low setting.
4. Once done, remove its lid of the crockpot carefully.

5.   Allow it to cool and refrigerate for 2 hour.

6.   Garnish as desired.

7.   Serve.

Walnut Balls

Ingredients:
- 4 tablespoons almond flour
- 2 teaspoon liquid stevia
- 2 fresh egg, beaten
- 2 oz walnuts, chopped
- 4 tablespoons butter
- 2 teaspoon baking powder
- 2 tablespoon Erythritol

Directions:

1.   Mix the chopped walnuts and butter.
2.   Add baking powder and Erythritol.
3.   Add almond flour, liquid stevia, and egg.
4.   Knead the dough until smooth.
5.   Make small balls from the dough.
6.   Cover the bottom of the slow cooker with the parchment and place the walnut balls inside.
7.   Cook the dessert for 4 hours on High.
8.   When the walnut balls are cooked, serve them immediately!

Cinnamon Cake

Ingredients:

- ¾ cup almond butter, melted
- 2 tablespoons Swerve
- 2 teaspoon baking soda
- 2 tablespoon lime juice
- 1 teaspoon almond extract
- 2 cup coconut flour
- 2 eggs, beaten
- 2 teaspoons ground cinnamon

Directions:

1.   In the mixing bowl combine the coconut flour with the fresh eggs and the other ingredients and whisk.
2.   Mix up the mixture well and transfer it in the slow cooker.
3.   Make the swirls with the help of the fork and close the lid.

4.   Cook the cake for 4 hours on High.

5.   Chill the cooked cake well and cut into the servings.

6.   After this, remove the cake from the slow cooker.

Coconut Bars

Ingredients:
- 2 fresh egg, beaten
- 2 teaspoon baking powder
- 2 teaspoon vanilla extract
- 2 cup coconut flour
- 2 tablespoons coconut flakes, unsweetened
- 4 tablespoons butter

Directions:
1. Mix the coconut flour and coconut flakes.
2. Add the butter and beaten egg.
3. Add baking powder and vanilla extract.
4. Stir the dough until smooth.
5. Place the dough in the slow cooker, press down to flatten and cook it for 2 hours on High.

6.   Cut the dessert into the bars and serve!

Almond Blondies

Ingredients:
- 2 teaspoon almond extract
- 2 cup almond flour
- 2 oz white chocolate, melted
- 1 cup almond butter, softened
- 2 cup stevia
- 2 fresh egg, beaten

Directions:

In the mixing bowl combine the butter with the stevia and the other ingredients and whisk.

1.   Line the crockpot with baking paper and pour blondies mixture inside.

2.   Flatten it and cook for 6 hours.

3.   Then remove the blondies from the crockpot and cut into the servings.

Spiced Strawberry Pudding

Ingredients:

- 2 tablespoon of apple pie spice
- 2 cups of almond flour
- 2 tablespoon of baking powder
- 2 fresh eggs
- 2 cups of strawberries, cored
- 2 tablespoon of vanilla

Directions:

1. Separately blend the wet and dry Ingredients: in the mixer.
2. Mix both the mixtures together in a bowl until smooth.
3. Now spread the cake batter in a greased ramekin and place it in the Crockpot.
4. Cover its lid and cook for 4 hours on Low setting.

5.   Once done, remove its lid of the crockpot carefully.

6.   Allow it to cool and refrigerate for 2 hour.

Chocolate Mousse

Ingredients:

*   2 cup almond milk, unsweetened
*   2 tablespoon full-fat cream cheese
*   2 oz dark chocolate
*   2 egg whites

Directions:

1.   Melt the chocolate and combine it with the almond milk.

2.   Whisk the egg whites until soft peaks and combine it together with the cream cheese.

3.   Whisk it gently for 2 minute more.

4.   Combine chocolate mixture and egg white mixture.

5.   Stir and transfer into ramekins.

6.   Place the ramekins in the slow cooker and cook on Low for 4 hours.

7.   Serve the cooked mousse!

Chocolate Pecan Cake

Ingredients:
- 2 teaspoon almond extract
- 2 tablespoons Stevia
- 2 teaspoon baking powder
- 1 oz dark chocolate, chopped
- 4 eggs, beaten
- 2 pecans, chopped
- Cooking spray
- 2 cup coconut flour
- 1/2 cup almond butter, melted
- 1/2 cup of water

Directions:

1. In a bowl mix the coconut flour with almond butter water and the other ingredients except the cooking spray.
2. Spray the slow cooker with cooking spray from inside and pour cake mixture.

3.   Flatten the surface of the cake mixture well and close the lid.

4.   Cook the spoon cake for 6 hours on Low.

Fresh Cream Mix

- 2 teaspoon cinnamon powder
- egg yolks
- tablespoons white sugar
- Zest of 2 orange, grated
- A pinch of nutmeg for serving
- tablespoons sugar
- cups water
- Preparation Time: 2 hour
- Cooking Time: 2 hour
- Servings: 6
- Ingredients:
- cups fresh cream

Directions:

1. In a bowl, mix cream, cinnamon and orange zest and stir.
2. In another bowl, mix the egg yolks with white sugar and whisk well.
3. Add this over the cream, stir, strain and divide into ramekins.

45

4. Put ramekins in your slow cooker, add 2 cups water to the slow cooker, cover, cook on Low for 2 hour, leave cream aside to cool down and serve.

Pears And Apples Bowls

Ingredients:

- 2 tablespoon walnuts, chopped
- tablespoons brown sugar
- 1 cup coconut cream
- 2 teaspoon vanilla extract
- pears, cored and cut into wedges
- apples, cored and cut into wedges

Directions:

1. In your slow cooker, mix the pears with the apples, nuts and the other ingredients, toss, put the lid on and cook on Low for 2 hours.
2. Divide the mix into bowls and serve cold.

Macadamia Fudge Truffles

Ingredients:

6 ounces dark chocolate, melted
2 tsp vanilla extract - 2 fresh egg, lightly beaten
2 cup roasted macadamia nuts, finely chopped
1 cup ground almonds - 2 ounces butter, melted

Directions:

1. Place the macadamia nuts, almonds, melted butter, melted chocolate, vanilla, and egg into a large bowl, stir until combined.
2. Grease the bottom of the crockpot by rubbing with butter.

3. Place the mixture into the crockpot and press down.
4. Set to cook low setting within 4 hours.
5. Allow the batter to cool until just warm.
6. Take a teaspoon, scoop the mixture out, and roll into balls.
7. Refrigerate to harden slightly. Store the truffle balls in the fridge.

Chocolate Covered Bacon Cupcakes

Ingredients:

2 tsp baking powder
2 eggs, lightly beaten
1 cup full-fat Greek yogurt

2 tsp vanilla extract

25 paper cupcake cases

6 slices streaky bacon, cut into small pieces, fried in a pan until crispy

6 ounces dark chocolate, melted

2 cup ground hazelnuts

Directions:

1. Mix the fried bacon pieces and melted chocolate in a bowl, set aside.
2. Mix the ground hazelnuts, baking powder, eggs, yogurt, vanilla, and a pinch of salt in a medium-sized bowl.
3. Spoon the hazelnut mixture into the cupcake cases.
4. Spoon the chocolate and bacon mixture on top of the hazelnut mixture.
5. Place the cupcake cases into the crockpot. Cook for 4 hours, high setting.

6. Remove the cupcakes from the pot and leave to cool on the bench before storing serving.
7. Serve with whipped cream!

Chocolate, Berry, And Macadamia Layered Jars

Ingredients:

- 8 ounces cream cheese
- 1 cup heavy cream
- 2 tsp vanilla extract
- 6 ounces dark chocolate, melted
- 1 cup mixed berries, (fresh) – any berries you like
- 1/3 cup toasted macadamia nuts, chopped

Directions:

1. Whisk the cream cheese, cream, and vanilla extract in a medium-sized bowl.
2. Scoop a small amount of melted chocolate, put it into each jar or ramekin.
3. Place a few berries on top of the chocolate.
4. Sprinkle some toasted macadamias onto the berries. Scoop the cream cheese mixture into the ramekin.
5. Place another layer of chocolate, berries, and macadamia nuts on top of the cream cheese mixture.
6. Put the jars inside the slow cooker and put the hot water until it reaches halfway up.
7. Set to low, then cook for 6 hours.
8. Remove the jars and leave them to cool and set on the bench for about 2 hours before serving.

Choco-Peanut Cake

Ingredients:

1 cup salted butter, melted
4 fresh eggs
8 oz. pkg. mini Reese's peanut butter cups
30 .26 oz. devil's food cake mix
2 cup of water
For the topping
4 Tbsp. powdered sugar
Ten bite-size Reese's peanut butter cups
2 cup creamy peanut butter

Directions:

1. Mix the cake mixture, ice, butter, and fresh eggs in a large bowl until smooth. Some lumps are all right, that's all right.

2. Cut the cups of the mini peanut butter. Cleaner non-stick spray on the slow cooker.
3. Add the butter slowly and spread over an even layer.
4. Cover and cook on high during the cooking time for 2 hours without opening the lid.
5. Melt the peanut butter over medium heat in a pan.
6. Stir until melted and smooth; observe as it burns hard.
7. To smooth, add the powdered sugar and whisk.
8. Pour over the butter of the sweetened peanut in the cake, then serve.

Crockpot Apple Pudding Cake

Ingredients:
- 2 cup milk
- 4 apples, diced
- 2 2 & /2 cups orange juice
- 1 cup honey
- 2 tbsp butter melted
- 2 tsp cinnamon
- 2 cups all-purpose flour
- 1/2 plus 1/2 cup sugar, divided
- 4 tsp baking powder
- 2 tsp salt
- 1 cup butter cold

Directions:

1. Mix the flour, 1/2 cup sugar, baking powder, and salt.
2. Slice the butter until you have coarse crumbs in the mixture.

55

3. Remove the milk from the crumbs until moistened.
4. Grease a 4 or 6 qt crockpot's bottom and sides.
5. Spoon the batter into the crockpot's bottom and spread evenly.
6. Place the diced apples evenly over the mixture.
7. Whisk together the orange juice, honey, butter, remaining sugar, and cinnamon in a medium-sized pan. Garnish the apples.
8. Place the crockpot opening with a clean kitchen towel, place the lid on, it prevents condensation from reaching the crockpot from the cover.
9. Place the crockpot on top and cook until apples are tender for 2 to 4 hours. Serve hot.

Crockpot Brownie Cookies

Ingredients:

- 1 c mini chocolate chips
- 1 c chopped walnuts optional
- 8 slices cookie dough slices
- One box brownie mix
- Two fresh eggs
- 1/2 c butter melted

Directions:

1. Combine your brownie mixture with butter, eggs, chocolate chips, and nuts.
2. Sprinkle with non-stick spray the inside of your crockpot.
3. Place eight slices of ready-made cookie dough or pile tbsp of it on the bottom.

4. In your slow cooker, pour brownie mixture on top and smooth out evenly. Put on the lid and cook on top for 2 hours.
5. To get both textures in your meal, scoop from the middle out to the edge for each serving.
6. If desired, serve warm for best results, top with ice cream.

Crockpot Chocolate Caramel Monkey Bread

Ingredients:

30 oz buttermilk biscuits
20 milk chocolate-covered caramels
1 tbsp sugar
1/2 tsp ground cinnamon

Directions:
1. Mix sugar and cinnamon and set aside.
2. Fill a parchment paper crockpot, cover up to the bottom.
3. Wrap 2 buttermilk biscuit dough around one chocolate candy to cover the candy completely, pinching the seam closed.
4. Place the biscuit-wrapped candy in the crockpot bottom, start in the

middle of the crockpot and work your way to the sides.

5. Continue to wrap candy and put it in the crockpot, leaving roughly 1 inch between each.
6. Repeat these steps with sweets wrapped in the second layer of biscuit.
7. Sprinkle the remaining cinnamon-sugar mixture on top when using all the dough and confectionery.
8. Cover the crockpot and cook for 5 hours on the lower side.
9. Once cooked, remove the lid and let cool slightly.
10. Use the edges of the parchment paper to lift the monkey bread out of the crockpot.
11. Allow cooling for at least 2 0-30 minutes.
12. Cut off any excess parchment paper around the edge when ready to serve.

13. In a shallow bread or bowl, put monkey bread and drizzle with chocolate and caramel sauces.

Slow Coocoffee Cake

Ingredients:

- 1 teaspoon baking soda
- One teaspoon ground cinnamon
- One teaspoon white vinegar
- One teaspoon salt - Two fresh eggs
- 1 cup chopped nuts optional
- 2 1 cups of all-purpose flour
- 2 & 1 cups of brown sugar
- 1/2 cup vegetable oil
- 4 cups almond milk
- Two teaspoons baking powder

Directions:

1. In a large bowl, whisk in flour, brown sugar, and salt. Remove the oil until it is crumbly mixed.
2. In the flour mixture, combine the baking powder, baking soda, and cinnamon with a wooden spoon or spatula.
3. In a measuring cup, place milk, oil, eggs, and vinegar and whisk until the fresh eggs are pounded, then add to the flour mixture and stir until mixed.
4. Spray a non-stick cooking spray 6 -8 Qt slow cooker or line with a slow cooker liner.
5. Pour into the crockpot with the batter.
6. Sprinkle the cake batter's nuts over the end.
7. Put a paper towel over the crockpot insert and place the lid on top of it.
8. Cook within 2 hour and 45 minutes, high s or 2 hours, and 45 minutes.

9. Serve warm directly from the crockpot or store for up to 4 days in an airtight container.

Slow Cooker Apple Pear Crisp

Ingredients:
Four apples, peeled and cut into 2 /2-inch slices
One tablespoon all-purpose flour
One tablespoon lemon juice
1 teaspoon ground cinnamon
1/2 teaspoon kosher salt
Pinch of ground nutmeg
4 Bosc pears, peeled and cut into 2 /2-inch slices
1/2 cup light brown sugar
For the Topping:
1/2 cup light brown sugar
1 teaspoon ground cinnamon

1 teaspoon kosher salt

1/3 cup all-purpose flour

1/3 cup old fashioned oats

1 cup chopped pecans

Eight tablespoons unsalted butter, cut into cubes

Directions:

1. Combine flour, oats, pecans, sugar, cinnamon, and salt to make the topping.
2. Press the butter into the dry fixing until it looks like coarse crumbs; set aside.
3. Coat lightly with a non-stick spray inside a 4-qt slow cooker: put apples and pears in the slow cooker. Add brown sugar, flour, juice of lemon, cinnamon, salt, and nutmeg.
4. Sprinkle with reserved topping, gently pressing the crumbs into the butter using your fingertips.

5. Layer the slow cooker with a clean dishtowel.

6. Cover and cook for 2-4 hours at low heat or 10 0 minutes at high temperature, remove the dishtowel and continue to cook, uncovered until the top is browned and apples are tender for about 2 hour. Serve cold.

Key Lime Dump Cake Recipe

Ingredients:
- 44 oz. Key Lime Pie Filling
- 8 tbsp. or 1 cup butter melted
- 30 .26 oz. Betty Crocker French Vanilla Cake Mix box

Directions:
1. Spray inside the Crock-Pot with a non-stick cooking spray.

2. Empty key lime pie cans filling in the Crock-Pot bottom and then spread evenly.
3. Mix the dry vanilla cake mix with the dissolved butter in a bowl.
4. Pour the crumble cake/butter mixture over the crockpot, spread evenly, and cover the crockpot with the lid.
5. Cook for 2 hours at high or 4 hours at low. serve with ice cream or whip cream.

Crockpot Cherry Dump Cake Recipe

Ingredients:
- 42 oz. Cherry Pie Filling
- 1 cup butter melted
- 30 .26 oz. Betty Crocker Devil's Food Cake Mix

Directions:

1. Spray with a non-stick cooking spray inside the crockpot.
2. Empty cherry pie filling cans into crockpot's bottom, then evenly spread out.
3. Combine dry cake mix with butter in a medium bowl. Pour the crumble cake/butter mixture over the crockpot plus cherries, scatter evenly, and cover the crockpot with a lid.
4. Cook for 2 hours at high, or 4 hours at low.
5. Use ice cream or whip cream to serve.

Crockpot Pumpkin Spice Cake Recipe

Ingredients:

1 cup Applesauce - Three fresh eggs

2 tsp. Pumpkin Pie Spice

30 .26 oz. Betty Crocker Spice Cake Mix

30 oz. Libby's Pure Pumpkin

Directions:

1. Whisk all the fixing with a mixer for 2 minute.
2. Spray with nonstick cooking spray inside the crockpot.
3. Pour over and cover the mixture into the crockpot.
4. Cook for 2 .6 – 2 hours or until finished. Serve.

Crockpot Blueberry Dump Cake Recipe

Ingredients:

42 oz. Blueberry Pie Filling

1 cup butter melted

30 .26 oz. Betty Crocker Lemon Cake Mix

Directions:

1. Spray with non-stick cooking spray the crockpot.
2. Put blueberry pie filling evenly into the bottom of the crockpot.
3. In a mixing bowl, combine dry lemon cake mix with melted butter and stir until crumbly.
4. Break some big chunks into the crumbles of a small spoon.
5. Pour the crumble cake/butter mixture over the blueberry mixture

into crockpot, spread evenly, and cover with a lid the crockpot.

6. Cook at high for 2 hours, and at low for 4 hours. Serve.

White Chocolate Fudge

Ingredients:

- 1/2 cup heavy whipping cream

- 1/2 cup honey

- 2 tsp vanilla

- 2 cups white chocolate, chopped

- 1 cup white chocolate chips

Directions:

1.   Add honey, heavy whipping cream, and white chocolate into the cooking pot and stir well.

2.   Cover instant pot aura with lid.

3.   Select slow cook mode and cook on HIGH for 2 hour.

4.   Cut into squares and serve.

Applesauce

Ingredients:

- 1/2 cup water
- 2 tsp ground cinnamon
- 25 medium apples, peeled, cored, and sliced
- 1/2 cup sugar

Directions:

1. Add all ingredients into the cooking pot and stir well.

2. Cover instant pot aura with lid.

3. Select slow cook mode and cook on LOW for 8 hours.

4. Transfer apple mixture into the blender and blend until smooth.

5. Serve and enjoy.

Delicious Bread Pudding

Ingredients:

- 4 cups of milk

- 1/3 cup maple syrup

- 2 tbsp cinnamon

- 6 fresh eggs

- 8 cups of bread cubes

- 2 tbsp vanilla

Directions:

1. In a large bowl, whisk together eggs, sugar, cinnamon, vanilla, and milk.

2. Add bread cubes into the cooking pot.

3. Pour egg mixture on top of bread cubes and let sit for 30 minutes.

4. Cover instant pot aura with lid.

5. Select slow cook mode and cook on LOW for 4 hours.

6. Serve and enjoy.

Rice Pudding

Ingredients:

- 1 tsp cinnamon

- 2 tsp vanilla

- 2 tbsp butter

- 1/2 tsp salt

- 1/3 cup long-grain rice

- 1/3 cup sugar

- 4 cups of milk

Directions:

1.   Add all ingredients into the cooking pot and stir well.

2.   Cover instant pot aura with lid.

3.   Select slow cook mode and cook on LOW for 4 hours.

4.   Stir well and serve.

Maple Pears

Ingredients:

- 2 tbsp ginger, sliced

- 2 cinnamon stick

- 6 cardamom pods

- 4 ripe pears, peel, core, and cut the bottom

- 1/2 cup maple syrup

- 2 cups orange juice

Directions:

1.   Place pears into the cooking pot.

2.   Mix together the remaining ingredients and pour over pears into the cooking pot.

3.   Cover instant pot aura with lid.

4. Select slow cook mode and cook on LOW for 4 hours.

5. Serve warm and enjoy.

Cinnamon Coconut Rice Pudding

Ingredients:

- 2 cups coconut cream

- 2 tsp ground cinnamon

- 2 tsp vanilla

- 2 cup rice, rinsed and uncooked

- 4 cups of coconut milk

Directions:

1.   Add all ingredients into the cooking pot and stir well.

2.   Cover instant pot aura with lid.

3.   Select slow cook mode and cook on LOW for 6 hours.

4.   Stir well and serve.

Fruit Compote

Ingredients:

- 25 oz apricots, dried
- 45 oz can peach, un-drained and sliced
- 25 oz can oranges, un-drained
- 25 Cherries
- 4 tbsp raisins
- 25 oz plums, dried

Directions:

1.   Add all ingredients into the cooking pot and stir well.

2.   Cover instant pot aura with lid.

3.   Select slow cook mode and cook on LOW for 6 hours.

4.   Stir well and serve.

Pumpkin Pie Pudding

Ingredients:

- 25 oz milk
- 30 oz can pumpkin
- 5 tsp vanilla extract
- 2 tsp pumpkin pie spice 2 eggs, beaten
- 2 tbsp butter, melted
- 1 cup biscuit mix
- 1/3 cup sugar
-

Directions:

1.   Add all ingredients into the cooking pot and mix well.

2.   Cover instant pot aura with lid.

3.   Select slow cook mode and cook on LOW for 6 hours.

4.   Serve with ice-cream and enjoy it.

Chocolate Almond Fudge

Ingredients:

- 2 tbsp almonds, sliced

- 2 tbsp swerve

- 2 tbsp butter, melted

- 8 oz chocolate chips

- 1 cup milk

Directions:

1.   Add chocolate chips, milk, butter, and swerve into the cooking pot and stir well.

2.   Cover instant pot aura with lid.

3.   Select slow cook mode and cook on LOW for 2 hours.

4.   Add almonds and stir fudge until smooth.

5.   Pour fudge mixture into the greased baking dish and spread evenly.

6.   Place baking dish in the refrigerator until the fudge set.

7.   Cut into squares and serve.

Delicious Chocolate Cake

Ingredients:

- 6 tbsp butter, melted
- 1 cup Swerve
- 2 cup almond flour
- Pinch of salt
- 4 large fresh eggs

- 2 1 tsp baking powder

- 4 tbsp whey protein powder

- 1 cup cocoa powder

- 1 tsp vanilla

- 1/2 cup almond milk

Directions:

1. Line instant pot aura cooking pot with parchment paper.

2. In a mixing bowl, whisk together almond flour, baking powder, protein powder, cocoa powder, swerve, and salt.

3. Stir in eggs, vanilla, almond milk, and butter until well combined.

4. Cover instant pot aura with lid.

5. Select slow cook mode and cook on LOW for 2 1 hours.

6. Serve and enjoy.

Shredded Coconut-Raspberry Cake

Ingredients:

- 2 teaspoons baking soda

- 1/2 teaspoon fine sea salt

- 4 large eggs, lightly beaten

- ¾ cup canned coconut milk

- 2 teaspoon coconut extract

- 2 cup raspberries, fresh or frozen

- 1 cup melted coconut oil, plus more for coating the slow cooker insert

- 2 cups almond flour

- 2 cup unsweetened shredded coconut

- 2 cup erythritol or 2 teaspoon stevia powder

- 1/2 cup unsweetened, unflavored protein powder

Directions:

1.   Generously coat the inside of the slow cooker insert with coconut oil.

2.   In a large bowl, stir together the almond flour, coconut, erythritol, protein powder, baking soda, and sea salt.

3.   Whisk in the eggs, coconut milk, 1 cup of coconut oil, and coconut extract.

4.   Gently fold in the raspberries.

5.   Transfer the batter to the prepared slow cooker, cover, and cook for 4 hours on low.

6.   Turn off the slow cooker and let the cake cool for several hours to room temperature.

7.   Serve at room temperature.

Poached Berries

Number of Servings: 4
Calories per Serving: 2 010

Ingredients:
- 1/2 cup frozen blueberries
- 1/2 cup frozen blackberries
- 1/2 cup fresh quartered strawberries
- 1 cup sucanat
- 5 cups water
- Juice of 1 lemon

Instructions:

1.   Combine the water, lemon juice, and sucanat in the slow cooker.

2.   Mix well.

3.   Add the berries and mix to coat in the sucanat mixture.

4.   Cover and cook for 4 hours on low, then serve warm or chilled.

Almond Chocolate Candy Bars

Ingredients:
- 2 cups chopped almonds
- 28 oz semisweet chocolate chips

Instructions:

1.   Combine the chocolate chips and chopped almonds in the slow cooker.

2.   Cover and cook for 2 hour on low, stirring once every 30 minutes.

3.   Spread out a sheet of wax paper and scoop the chocolate and almond mixture onto it.

4.   Spread out thinly with a spatula.

5.   Let the mixture stand for at least 20 minutes to harden, then divide into 2 8 even pieces.

6.   Place in a tightly sealed jar and keep refrigerated.

Carrot Cake

Ingredients:
- 1 6 tsp grated nutmeg
- 2 /8 tsp ground cloves
- 1 cup grated carrots
- 2 Tbsp water
- 1/2 cup chopped walnuts
- Nonstick cooking spray
- 2 large egg or 2 mashed banana
- 2 Tbsp butter
- 1/2 cup sucanat
- 1/3 cup all-purpose flour
- 1 tsp baking powder
- 1/2 tsp baking soda
- 1/2 tsp cinnamon

Instructions:

1.   In a bowl, combine the baking soda, flour, baking powder, cinnamon, nutmeg, cloves, and salt.

2.   In the food processor, combine the butter, sucanat, and egg or banana. Pulse until creamy, then mix into the flour mixture.

3.   Stir the water and carrots into the batter, then fold in the nuts.

4.   Coat the inside of the slow cooker with the nonstick cooking spray, then pour the batter into it. Spread the mixture evenly using a spatula.

5.   Cover and cook for 2 hours on low, or until the cake becomes firm.

6.   Poke the center with a toothpick; if it comes out clean, it is ready to be eaten.

Indian Pudding

Ingredients:
- 1 cup dark molasses
- 1 cup cornmeal
- 2 /8 tsp baking soda
- 1/2 cup mashed banana
- 4 cups heated milk
- 2 Tbsp sucanat
- 2 Tbsp unsalted butter

Instructions:

1.   In a saucepan over medium flame, combine 5 cups of heated milk with all of the other ingredients.

2.   Bring to a boil, then stir in the remaining milk.

3.   Transfer the mixture into the slow cooker, then cover and cook for 4 hours on low.

4.   Divide into 6 equal pieces before serving to control the calorie content per serving.

Simple Applesauce

Ingredients:

● 2 Tbsp freshly squeezed lemon juice
● 4 inches cinnamon stick
● 6 medium apples, peeled, cored, and chopped
● 2 Tbsp water

Instructions:

1.   Combine the apples, lemon juice, cinnamon stick, and water in the slow cooker.

2.   Cover and cook for 4 hours on low, or until the apples become extra tender.

3.   Use a fork or a potato masher to mash the applesauce to a desired consistency.

4.   For smooth applesauce, use an immersion blender or food processor.

5.   Serve over gluten free bread. Refrigerate in a tightly sealed container for up to 2 weeks.

6.   Add sucanat to sweeten the applesauce, but this would increase the calories per cup.

Caramel And Bread Pudding

Ingredients:
- 1/2 cup sucanat
- 1 tsp vanilla
- 1 cup caramel topping
- 6 oz sweet bread, cubed
- 1/2 cup mashed banana
- 2 cups skim milk

Instructions:

1.   Spread the bread cubes in the slow cooker insert.

2.   In a bowl, beat the banana, milk, sucanat, and vanilla, then pour on top of the bread cubes.

3.   Press down on the mixture with a ladle.

4.   Cover and refrigerate for 4 hours or more.

5.   Place the insert into the slow cooker and let stand for 30 minutes to thaw slightly.

6.   Cover and cook for 6 hours on low.

7.   Divide into six equal servings to control calorie content per serving. Divide the caramel topping evenly over each serving, then serve.

Caramel Apples And Pears

Ingredients:
- 8 oz package of caramels
- 1/2 cup apple juice
- 1 tsp cinnamon
- 2 green apple, cored and peeled
- 2 pear, cored and peeled
- 2 Tbsp butter

Instructions:

1. Slice the apples and pears into wedges.

2. In the slow cooker, combine the apple juice, butter, cinnamon, and caramels.

3. Cover and cook for 2 hour on low, or until everything is melted.

4. Mix well.

5.   Add the apple and pear wedges, then turn to coat in the mixture. Cover and cook for 2 hour on low, or until fruits are fork tender. Serve warm.

Glazed Bananas

Ingredients:
- 2 Tbsp sucanat
- 2 Tbsp coconut rum
- 1 tsp vanilla
- 4 large bananas, just ripe
- 2 Tbsp unsalted butter, softened
- 2 Tbsp freshly squeezed lime juice

Instructions:

1. Peel the bananas and slice them in half lengthwise.

2. Coat the bottom of the slow cooker with the softened butter, then place the halved bananas with the cut sides facing down, in the slow cooker in a single layer.

3. In a bowl, mix together the vanilla, sucanat, rum, and lime juice.

4. Pour the mixture all over the bananas.

5. Cover and cook for 2 hours on low. Serve warm.

Apple Cake

Ingredients:

- 2 tsp cinnamon
- 1/3 cup sucanat
- 4 apples, peeled, cored and chopped
- Non-stick cooking spray
- 1/2 cup mashed banana
- 2 cup almond flour
- 2 tsp baking powder
- 2 tsp vanilla

Instructions:

1. Coat the inside of the slow cooker with nonstick cooking spray.

2. In a bowl, combine the flour, baking powder, sucanat, and cinnamon.

3. Stir in the chopped apples to coat in the mixture.

4. Combine the mashed banana and vanilla, then mix it in with the flour

mixture. Add just enough water to moisten the batter, if needed.

5.   Transfer the mixture into the slow cooker. Cover and cook for 2 hours and 45 minutes on high.

6.   Divide the cake into equal servings to control the calories per serving.

7.   Best served warm.

Fruit Granola

Ingredients:
- 2 tsp cinnamon
- 4 apples, cored and diced
- 6 0 g sultanas
- 6 0 g unsalted butter, melted
- Non-stick cooking spray
- 2 00 g oatmeal
- 6 00 g plain granola meal
- 2 Tbsp raw honey
- 1 tsp nutmeg

Instructions:

1. Coat the inside of the slow cooker with nonstick cooking spray.

2. Combine the melted butter and honey in one bowl.

3. Combine the oatmeal, granola meal, cinnamon, apples, and sultanas in another bowl.

4.   Gradually mix in the butter and honey until mixture is moist.

5.   Transfer the mixture into the slow cooker.

6.   Cover and cook for 2 hours on low.

7.   Divide the mixture into five equal servings to control the number of calories per serving.

8.   Store in an airtight container. Serve with milk, if desired.

Pumpkin Pudding

Ingredients:
- 1/2 cup mashed banana
- 2 tsp pumpkin pie spice
- 1 tsp lemon peel
- Non-stick cooking spray
- 8 oz unsweetened pumpkin
- 2 Tbsp sucanat
- 2 Tbsp almond flour
- 1/3 cup fat free evaporated milk

Instructions:

1. Coat the inside of the slow cooker with nonstick cooking spray.

2. Combine the pumpkin, sucanat, flour, milk, banana, pumpkin pie spice, and lemon peel in a bowl. Mix well.

3. Pour the batter into the slow cooker, then cover and cook for 2 hours on low. Serve chilled or warm.

Fruitcake

Ingredients:

- 4 oz candied cherries, halved
- 4 oz mixed candied fruit
- 2 cup slivered almonds
- 1 tsp almond extract
- 1 tsp vanilla extract
- Non-stick cooking spray
- 5 cups flour
- 1/2 cup pineapple juice
- 2 cup unsweetened crushed pineapple, drained
- 5 tsp baking powder
- 1 cup softened unsalted butter
- 4 eggs, separated
- 2 cup sucanat
- 5 cups golden raisins

Instructions:

1.   Coat a cake pan with nonstick cooking spray.

2.   Beat the butter and sucanat until creamy using an electric mixer.

3.   Add the yolks and mix well.

4.   In a bowl, combine the baking powder and flour, then add gradually into the yolk mixture, alternating between it and the pineapple juice.

5.   Fold the raisins, crushed pineapple, candied fruit, and extract into the batter.

6.   In a separate bowl, whip the egg whites until stiff, then fold into the batter.

7.   Pour the mixture into the prepared cake pan and cover with aluminum foil.

8.   Place the pan on a rack in the slow cooker and pour about half a cup of warm water around the pan.

9.   Cover and cook for 4 hours on high.

10.   Set aside to rest for 25 minutes before removing the cake.

11.   Set aside to cool before slicing.

12.   Slice evenly into 30 servings to control calories per serving.

Simple Custard

Ingredients:

- 1 tsp brown sugar
- 1/2 tsp cinnamon
- Nonstick cooking spray
- 1/2 cup sucanat
- 2 cups skim milk
- 1/3 cup mashed banana

Instructions:

1.   Grease a baking dish that can fit inside the slow cooker using nonstick cooking spray.

2.   Pour the milk into a saucepan and place over medium flame.

3.   Cook until a skin starts to form, then turn off the heat and set aside.

4.   In a bowl, mix together the vanilla, mashed banana, and sucanat.

5.   Gradually mix in the cooled skim milk.

6.   Transfer the mixture into the prepared baking dish.

7.   Combine the cinnamon and brown sugar in a bowl then sprinkle the mixture on top of the custard.

8.   Cover the baking dish with aluminum foil, then place it on a rack in the slow cooker.

9.   Carefully pour hot water around the dish until it is about an inch above the base of the cooker.

10.   Cover and cook for 4 hours on high or until the custard is set.

11.   Slice into equal servings and serve warm.

Raspberry Peach Cobbler

Ingredients:
- 1/2 cup toasted sliced almonds
- 1/2 cup oat flour
- 1 tsp ground cloves
- 2 tsp ground cinnamon
- 2 tsp vanilla
- 4 Tbsp chopped unsalted butter
- Salt
- Nonstick cooking spray
- 280g fresh raspberries or 25 oz frozen, thawed and drained
- 2 1 lb fresh ripe peaches or 4 2 oz frozen thawed, and drained
- 5 Tbsp quick cooking tapioca
- 1/2 cup frozen orange juice concentrate, thawed
- 1 cup and 2 Tbsp sucanat, divided
- 1/2 cup rolled oats

Instructions:

1.   Coat the inside of the slow cooker with nonstick cooking spray.

2.   Pour the peaches and raspberries into the slow cooker.

3.   In a cup, mix together the orange juice concentrate and tapioca.

4.   Pour the mixture over the peaches and raspberries.

5.   Combine 2 teaspoon of cinnamon, 1/2 cup of sucanat, and the zest, vanilla, and cloves in a bowl.

6.   Pour the mixture into the slow cooker and mix everything well.

7.   In a bowl, mix together the oats, remaining sucanat and cinnamon, and the almonds, flour, butter, and salt.

8. Mix well until crumbly, then sprinkle on top of the fruit mixture in the slow cooker.

9. Cover and cook for 2 hours on high. Divide equally into eight servings to control the calories per serving.

Low Cal Chocolate Cake

Ingredients:

- 1/2 cup mashed banana
- 2 tsp baking soda
- 1 tsp vanilla
- 1 cup buttermilk
- Nonstick cooking spray
- 2 oz unsweetened chocolate
- 2 Tbsp unsalted butter
- 4 cups flour
- 1/2 cup sucanat

Instructions:

1. Coat two vegetable cans with nonstick cooking spray and set aside.

2. Melt and cool the unsweetened chocolate, then set aside.

116

3.   In a bowl, beat the butter and sucanat together using an electric mixer.

4.   Add the mashed banana and mix well.

5.   Add the chocolate and mix well.

6.   Combine the flour and baking soda in a separate bowl, then gradually beat it into the butter mixture, alternating with the vanilla and buttermilk.

7.   Mix everything well.

8.   Pour the mixture into the prepared vegetable cans, then seal with aluminum foil.

9.   Place the cans into the slow cooker, then pour half a cup of warm water around the cans.

10.   Cover the slow cooker and cook for 2 hour and 45 minutes on high.

11. Carefully take the cans out of the cooker and set aside for 25 minutes before removing from the cans.

12. Slice into eight equal servings to control the amount of calories per serving.

Baked Green Apple And Raisin Delight

Ingredients:

- 1/2 cup honey
- 4 Tbsp coconut oil
- 1 tsp cinnamon
- 4 large green apples
- 4 Tbsp raisins

Instructions:

1. Remove the core from the apples, but make sure to leave the bottom untouched.

2. In a bowl, combine the coconut oil, honey, cinnamon and raisins.

3. Spoon the mixture into the apples and arrange them in the slow cooker.

4.   Pour about 1 inch of water into the slow cooker, cover, and cook for 8 hours on low.

5.   Carefully remove the baked apples using a pair of tongs and arrange on a platter.

6.   Serve warm.

Date Pudding

Ingredients:

- 2 tsp coconut butter
- 2 tsp ground cinnamon
- 2 Tbsp coconut powder
- Coconut oil
- 1 cup chopped dates
- 6 cups water
- 2 cups oats, gluten free

Instructions:

1. Grease the slow cooker with coconut oil then combine the butter, dates, oats, coconut powder, cinnamon and water in it.

2. Cover and cook for 6 hours on low.

3. Remove the pudding from the slow cooker with a spatula, then slice and serve.

Nutty Maple Apple

Ingredients:

- 1/2 cup high quality maple syrup
- 1/2 cup apple cider
- 5 tsp ground cinnamon
- 6 medium apples
- 1/2 cup dried cherries
- 1/2 cup chopped walnuts

Instructions:

1.   Remove the core from the apples, but make sure to leave the bottoms intact.

2.   Place in the slow cooker.

3.   In a bowl, mix together the cherries and walnuts.

4.   Sprinkle the cinnamon all over and toss to coat.

5.   Spoon the mixture into the cored apples.

6.   Pour the maple syrup on top of the apples, then pour the apple cider into the slow cooker around the apples.

7.   Cover and cook for 2 hours on low.

8.   Turn off the heat, take off the lid and let stand for 25 minutes.

9.   Arrange apples on a platter and spoon the sauce over each.

10.   Excess can be placed in a leak-proof container in the refrigerator for up to 8 2 hours.

Peanut Butter And Chocolate Cake

Ingredients:

- 1 tsp baking powder
- 5 Tbsp melted coconut butter
- 2 cup boiling water
- 2 Tbsp chopped almonds
- 2 Tbsp melted peanut butter
- Nonstick cooking spray
- 1/3 cup almond flour
- 1 cup creamy peanut butter
- 1/2 cup coconut flakes
- 1/2 cup unsweetened cocoa powder
- 1/2 cup sour cream
- 1/2 cup coconut sugar
- 1 tsp almond extract
- 1 tsp baking soda

Instructions:

1.   Grease the slow cooker with non-stick cooking spray.

2.   Combine the sugar, flour, baking powder, and baking soda in a bowl then stir in the sour cream and peanut butter.

3.   Stir in the melted coconut butter and almond extract until you get a thick batter.

4.   Pour the batter into the slow cooker.

5.   In another bowl, combine the coconut flakes with the coconut powder and then add the boiling water as you stir to make a smooth mixture.

6.   Pour the mixture on top of the batter inside the slow cooker.

7.   Cover the slow cooker and cook for 4 hours on low or until the cake becomes firm.

8.   Poke the center with a toothpick to check. If it comes out clean, it is ready.

9.   Loosen the cake from the slow cooker and turn over onto a platter.

10.   Drizzle the melted peanut butter on top and sprinkle with almonds.

11. Set aside to cool for about 25 minutes.

Rhubarb And Raspberry Crunch

Ingredients:

- A dash of salt
- Nonstick cooking spray
- 6 cups chopped rhubarb
- 6 cups raspberries
- 5 cups gluten free oats
- 1/2 cup brown sugar
- 5 Tbsp tapioca
- 3 cup almond flour
- 1/2 cup coconut butter
- 1/2 tsp ground ginger
- 4 tsp cinnamon

Instructions:

1. Cover the slow cooker with non-stick cooking spray and combine the

rhubarb, raspberries, brown sugar, tapioca, cinnamon and ginger in it.

2.   Mix well to combine.

3.   Cover and cook for half an hour on medium.

4.   Combine the oats, butter and flour in a bowl using clean, dry hands to make crumbs.

5.   Sprinkle the crumbs into the slow cooker.

6.   Cover and cook on low for 4 hours or until the rhubarb becomes very tender.

7.   Spoon the mixture onto a platter and set aside to cool then serve.

Dulce De Leche

Ingredients:

- 4 small cans of sweetened condensed milk

Instructions:

1. Thoroughly remove the labels from the canned condensed milk.

2. Do not puncture or open in any way.

3. Place the cans inside the slow cooker and pour just enough water to submerge the cans about three quarters of the way.

4. Cover and cook for 6 hours on high.

5. Remove the cans from the slow cooker using a pair of tongs and set aside to cool completely.

6. Open up the cans and using a rubber spatula, transfer into clean, dry containers with a tight lid.

7. Refrigerate for at least half an hour before serving.

Mango Oatmeal

Ingredients:

- 2 cups coconut milk
- 2 cups mango, sliced
- 2 tsp cinnamon
- 2 tsp cardamom
- 2 tsp salt
- 2 tsp vanilla extract
- 1 cup coconut oil or organic butter
- 4 cups oats, gluten free
- 2 Tbsp apple cider vinegar
- 6 cups water
- 1 cup honey

Instructions:

1.   The day before, rub the coconut oil or butter all over the slow cooker, then stir in the oats, water, and apple cider vinegar.

2.   Cover and let soak for 25 hours, unplugged.

3.   Stir in the mango, cardamom, cinnamon, salt, and vanilla extract.

4.   Set the slow cooker on low and cook for 8 hours.

5.   Right before serving, stir in the coconut milk and honey.

6.   Ladle into bowls and serve piping hot.

Pumpkin Pie Oatmeal

Ingredients:

- 2 tsp vanilla extract
- 2 tsp nutmeg
- 2 Tbsp maple syrup or honey or apple sauce
- 2 cups non fat Greek yogurt

- 2 cups oats, gluten free
- 8 cups water
- 2 cups unsweetened or homemade pumpkin puree
- 2 Tbsp coconut oil or organic butter
- 2 tsp cinnamon

Instructions:

1.   Rub the coconut oil or butter all over the slow cooker then combine the oats and water in it.

2.   Cover and let soak for about 25 hours, unplugged.

3.   Do not drain.

4.   Stir the pumpkin puree, cinnamon, nutmeg, vanilla extract, and maple syrup or honey or applesauce into the slow cooker.

5.   Cover and cook for 4 hours on high or for 8 hours on low.

6.   Ladle into bowls and top with yogurt and an extra dash of nutmeg, if desired.

Broccoli And Quinoa Casserole

Ingredients:

- 4 cups quinoa
- 2 cups broccoli florets, roughly chopped
- 2 cups sweet peppers, sliced
- 6 cloves garlic, minced
- 4 cups tomato paste, gluten free
- 6 to 8 cups water
- Optional: 2 cups goat cheese

Instructions:

1.   Combine the garlic, pepper, broccoli, and quinoa in the slow cooker.

2.   Pour the tomato paste on top, followed by just enough water to cover all of the ingredients.

3.   Cover and cook for 8 hours on low.

4.   Spoon onto serving plates and top with goat cheese.

Chicken Sausage And Sweet Potato Hash

Ingredients:

- 1/2 cup chicken broth
- 2 medium white fresh onion, diced
- 6 large sweet potatoes, peeled and grated
- 4 firm apples, peeled, cored, and diced
- 5 lb chicken sausage

Instructions:

1.   Remove the sausage from the casings, then place the sausage in a bowl and crumble with a fork or with your fingers.

2.   Add the grated sweet potatoes into the sausage and mix well.

3.   Add the onion and apples and mix again.

4.   Transfer the mixture into the slow cooker and pack firmly.

5.   Pour the broth on top.

6.   Cover and cook for 8 hours on low or for 4 hours on high.

7.   Serve warm, preferably with poached eggs.

Blueberry Slow Cooker Cake

Ingredients:

- 2 cup coconut or maple sugar
- 2 tsp vanilla extract
- A dash of salt
- Optional: lemon zest, as needed
- 4 cups blueberries
- 2 cups milk
- 2 cup almond flour
- 2 cup rice flour or gluten free pancake mix
- 4 fresh eggs
- 4 Tbsp coconut oil or organic butter

Instructions:

1.   Rub the coconut oil or organic butter all over the slow cooker, then lightly coat with the almond flour.

2.   Pour in the blueberries.

3.   In a bowl, whisk the fresh eggs together with the salt, sugar, and rice flour or pancake mix until smooth.

4.   Stir in the vanilla extract and milk and mix until smooth.

5.   Pour the battcr into the slow cooker on top of the berries.

6.   Sprinkle with lemon zest.

7.   Cover the slow cooker and cook for 4 hours on low, checking to see if the edges have browned and cake is puffed and set.

8.   Otherwise, add another hour of cooking time on low.

9.   Remove the cake from the slow cooker and place on a platter.

10. Slice and serve with honey, if desired.

Vegetable Frittata

Ingredients:

- 1/3 cup unflavored almond milk
- 1/3 tsp freshly ground black pepper
- 5 tsp olive oil
- 30 large fresh eggs
- 2 large white fresh onion, diced
- 1/3 cup diced green bell pepper
- 1/3 cup diced red bell pepper
- 5 tsp sea salt
- 5 cups sliced white mushrooms
- 1/3 tsp ground cumin

Instructions:

1.   Beat the fresh eggs in a large bowl, then mix in the almond milk.

2.   Season with salt, pepper, and cumin. Mix well.

3.   Stir the fresh onion, mushrooms, and bell peppers into the mixture. Set aside.

4.   Rub the olive oil all over the inside of the slow cooker using a cotton ball.

5.   Add the egg mixture in.

6.   Cover and cook for 8 hours on low.

7.   Serve warm, preferably with gluten free muffins.

Ham And Greens Casserole

Ingredients:

- 2 cup diced mushrooms
- 2 cups baby spinach
- 2 cups shredded Jack cheese
- 2 tsp garlic powder
- 2 tsp salt
- Non-stick cooking spray or coconut oil or butter
- 8 fresh eggs
- 2 cups diced ham
- 2 cup non-fat Greek yogurt
- 1 cup milk

Instructions:

1.   Grease the slow cooker using the non-stick cooking spray or coconut oil or butter.

2. Beat the fresh eggs in a bowl then beat in the milk, yogurt, garlic powder, and salt until thoroughly combined.

3. Mix in the mushrooms, cheese, spinach, and ham until well distributed.

4. Pour the egg mixture into the slow cooker.

5. Cover, set on medium heat and cook for 4 hours, or until the fresh eggs have set.

6. If still runny at the end of cooking time, cook for an additional hour on low.

7. Remove the casserole from the slow cooker and place on a plate.

8. Slice and serve warm.

Vanilla Chocolate Walnut Fudge

Ingredients:

- 2 teaspoons stevia powder

- 1/2 teaspoon fine sea salt

- 2 teaspoons pure vanilla extract

- 2 cup chopped toasted walnuts

- Coconut oil for coating the slow cooker insert and a baking dish

- 2 cup canned coconut milk

- 4 ounces unsweetened chocolate, chopped

- 2 cup erythritol

Directions

1.   Generously coat the inside of the slow cooker insert with coconut oil.

2. In a large bowl, whisk the coconut milk into a uniform consistency.

3. Add the chocolate, erythritol, stevia powder, and sea salt.

4. Stir to mix well.

5. Pour into the slow cooker. Cover and cook for 2 hours on low.

6. When finished, stir in the vanilla.

7. Let the fudge sit in the slow cooker, with the lid off, until it cools to room temperature, about 4 hours.

8. Coat a large baking dish with coconut oil and set aside.

9. Stir the fudge until it becomes glossy, about 25 minutes.

10. Stir in the walnuts.

11. Transfer the mixture to the prepared baking dish and smooth it into an even layer with a rubber spatula.

12. Refrigerate overnight.

13. Serve chilled, cut into small pieces.

Delicious Chocolate Peanut Butter Fudge

Ingredients:

• 2 teaspoon pure vanilla extract

• 4 ounces unsweetened chocolate, chopped

• 1 cup erythritol

• 2 teaspoon stevia powder

• Coconut oil for coating the slow cooker insert

• 2 1 cups heavy (whipping) cream

• 2 cup all-natural peanut butter

• 2 tablespoon unsalted butter, melted

Directions:

1.   Generously coat the inside of the slow cooker insert with coconut oil.

2.   In the slow cooker, stir together the heavy cream, peanut butter, butter, vanilla, chocolate, erythritol, and stevia.

3.   Cover and cook for 2 hours on low, stirring occasionally.

4.   Line a small, rimmed baking sheet with parchment or wax paper.

5.   Transfer the cooked fudge to the prepared sheet and refrigerate for at least 4 hours.

6.   Cut into squares and serve chilled.

White Chocolate Fudge

Ingredients:

- 1/2 cup heavy whipping cream
- 1/2 cup honey
- 2 tsp vanilla
- 2 cups white chocolate, chopped
- 1 cup white chocolate chips

Directions:

1.   Add honey, heavy whipping cream, and white chocolate into the cooking pot and stir well.

2.   Cover instant pot aura with lid.

3.   Select slow cook mode and cook on HIGH for 2 hour.

4.   Pour melted chocolate into the parchment-lined baking dish and place it in the fridge until set.

5.   Cut into squares and serve.

Delicious Bread Pudding

Ingredients:

- 4 cups of milk

- 1/3 cup maple syrup

- 2 tbsp cinnamon

- 6 fresh eggs

- 8 cups of bread cubes

- 2 tbsp vanilla

Directions:

1.   In a large bowl, whisk together eggs, sugar, cinnamon, vanilla, and milk.

2.   Add bread cubes into the cooking pot.

3.   Pour egg mixture on top of bread cubes and let sit for 30 minutes.

4.   Cover instant pot aura with lid.

5.   Select slow cook mode and cook on LOW for 4 hours.

Vanilla Pudding

Ingredients:

- 1 tsp cinnamon
- 2 tsp vanilla
- 2 tbsp butter
- 1/2 tsp salt
- 1/3 cup Vanilla
- 1/3 cup sugar
- 4 cups of milk

Directions:

1.   Add all ingredients into the cooking pot and stir well.

2.   Cover instant pot aura with lid.

3.   Select slow cook mode and cook on LOW for 4 hours.

4.   Stir well and serve.

Delightful Crème Brule

Ingredients:

- 1 tablespoon of cocoa powder
- 1 cup of swerve
- 1/2 cup of superfine swerve
- 6 egg yolks
- 2 cups of heavy cream
- 2 tablespoon of vanilla extract

Directions:
1. Start by thoroughly blending all the Ingredients: in a blender until smooth.
2. Now divide the batter into 4 ramekins and place them in the Crockpot.
3. Cover its lid and cook for 2 hours on Low setting.
4. Once done, remove its lid of the crockpot carefully.
5. Allow it to cool and refrigerate for 2 hour.

6. Serve.

Blueberry Crisp

Ingredients:

- 2 teaspoon almond extract
- ¾ teaspoon ground nutmeg
- 2 tablespoon Erythritol
- 2 fresh egg, beaten
- 1 cup blueberries
- 1/2 cup coconut flakes
- 2 tablespoons almond butter, softened

Directions:

1. In the mixing bowl, combine the berries with the flakes and the other ingredients and whisk.
2. Put the homogenous berries mixture in the crockpot and flatten well.
3. Flatten the crisp gently.

4. Close the lid.
5. Cook the crisp 6 hours on Low.

Almond Spread

Ingredients:

- 2 tablespoons cocoa powder
- 1 teaspoon almond extract
- 1/2 cup stevia
- 2 cup almond butter
- 1/2 cup almonds, chopped

Directions:

1. In the crockpot, mix the almonds with almond butter and the other ingredients and whisk
2. Close the lid and the mixture for 45 minutes in High.
3. Then whisk the mixture with the help of the hand mixer/blender.
4. Divide into bowls and serve.

Cinnamon Almonds

Ingredients:

- 2 teaspoons of vanilla
- 4 cups of almonds
- ⅛ cup of water
- 2 cup of brown swerve
- 4 tablespoons of cinnamon ground
- ⅛ teaspoon of salt
- 2 egg white

Directions:

1. Start putting all the Ingredients: into the Crockpot.
2. Cover its lid and cook for 4 hours on Low setting with occasional stirring
3. Once done, remove the pot's lid and give it a stir.
4. Serve fresh.

Pumpkin Custard

Ingredients:

- 2 teaspoon of pumpkin spice
- 2 pinch salt
- 1/2 teaspoon of cinnamon ground
- 2 cup of heavy cream
- Walnuts, to serve
- 2 cup of pumpkin puree
- 6 fresh eggs
- 1/3 cup of brown swerve

Directions:

1. Start by blending all the Ingredients: together in a mixer.
2. Pour this mixture into 4 ramekins and place them in the Crockpot.
3. Cover its lid and cook for 4 hours on Low setting.
4. Once done, remove its lid of the crockpot carefully.

5. Allow it to cool and refrigerate for 2 hour.
6. Garnish with walnuts and cream.
7. Serve.
8. Serve.

Almond Cocoa Cake

Ingredients:

- Pinch of salt
- 4 large fresh eggs
- 2 teaspoon vanilla
- 1 cup dark chocolate chips
- ¾ cup butter, melted
- 2 1 cups powdered sweetener
- ⅔ cup Dutch cocoa powder
- ⅓ cup ground almonds

Directions:

1. Line the crock-pot with aluminium foil and butter it.
2. In a bowl, mix all the ingredients.
3. Pour the batter into the buttered crock-pot.
4. Cover the pot with a paper towel to absorb the water.
5. Cover, cook on low for 4 hours.

Raspberry Tart

Ingredients:

- 2 cup raspberries
- 4 tablespoons coconut flour
- 4 tablespoons butter
- 4 tablespoons Erythritol
- 2 teaspoon vanilla extract
- 2 teaspoon ground ginger

Directions:

1. Combine butter, coconut flour, ground ginger, and vanilla extract.
2. Knead the dough.
3. Cover the bottom of the slow cooker with parchment.
4. Place the dough in the slow cooker and flatten it to the shape of a pie crust.
5. Place the raspberries over the piecrust and sprinkle with Erythritol.
6. Cook the tart for 4 hours on High.
7. Serve the cooked tart chilled.

Keto Sweet Bread

Ingredients:

- 1/2 cup almond milk
- 4 tablespoons butter
- 2 oz pumpkin seeds
- 2 cup coconut flour
- 1/2 cup Erythritol
- 2 teaspoon baking powder

Directions:

1. Mix the coconut flour and Erythritol.
2. Add the baking powder and almond milk.
3. Add butter and stir it gently.
4. Add the pumpkin seeds and knead the dough.
5. Place the dough in the slow cooker and cook the bread for 4 hours on High.
6. Slice the cooked bread and enjoy!

Coconut Bars

Ingredients:

- 2 teaspoon baking powder
- 2 teaspoon vanilla extract
- 2 teaspoon butter
- 1/2 cup coconut flakes, unsweetened
- 2 cup coconut flour
- 1 cup almond milk, unsweetened

Directions:

1. Mix the coconut flakes and coconut flour.
2. Add the baking soda and stir the mixture.
3. Add the butter and vanilla extract.
4. Add the almond milk and stir it until smooth.
5. Transfer the mixture to the slow cooker.
6. Flatten it with a spatula and cook for 4 hours on High.

7. Cut the cooked dessert into bars and serve!

Spoon Cake

Ingredients:

- 2 tablespoon butter
- 2 oz dark chocolate
- 2 tablespoons Erythritol
- 2 teaspoon ground cinnamon
- 1 cup almond milk, unsweetened
- 2 teaspoon baking powder
- 2 cup almond flour

Directions:

1. Mix the baking powder, almond milk, almond flour, butter, Erythritol, and ground cinnamon.
2. Chop the chocolate.
3. Stir the flour mixture until smooth, add the chopped chocolate.
4. Stir and transfer in the slow cooker.

5. Cook the cake for 2 hours on High.
6. Let the cake cool for 25 minutes and serve!

Berry & Coconut Cake

Ingredients:

- 2 large fresh egg, beaten with a fork
- 1/2 cup coconut flour
- 1/2 cup coconut milk
- 2 Tablespoons coconut oil
- 4 cups fresh or frozen blueberries and raspberries
- 2 Tablespoon butter for greasing the crock
- 2 cup almond flour
- ¾ cup sweetener of your choice
- 2 teaspoon baking soda
- 1/2 teaspoon salt

Directions:

1. Butter the crock-pot well.
2. In a bowl, whisk the fresh egg, coconut milk, and oil together.
3. Mix the dry ingredients.
4. Slowly stir in the wet ingredients.
5. Do not over mix.
6. Pour the batter in the crock-pot, spread evenly.
7. Spread the berries on top.
8. Cover, cook on high for 2 hours.
9. Cool in the crock for 2 -2 hours.

Almond Roll

Ingredients:

- 2 tablespoons stevia
- 1/2 cup coconut oil
- 2 teaspoon almond extract
- 2 fresh egg, beaten
- ¾ cup Mascarpone cream
- 2 teaspoon baking powder
- 2 cup almond flour
- 2 tablespoon ground cinnamon

Directions:

1. In a bowl mix the flour with coconut oil and the other ingredients except the cinnamon and stevia.
2. Mix up together ground cinnamon with stevia
3. Roll up the dough with the help of the rolling pin.

4. Spread the surface of the dough with ground cinnamon mixture and roll it into the log.
5. Cut the log into 6 buns and secure the edges of every bun.
6. Line the crockpot with baking paper.
7. Place the buns in the crockpot and close the lid.
8. Cook the cinnamon roll for 5 hours on High.
9. Check if the rolls are cooked with the help of the toothpick – if it is dry, the buns are cooked.
10. Chill the dessert well and then remove from the crockpot in the serving plate.

Red Velvet Cupcakes

Ingredients:

- 2 teaspoon vanilla extract
- 1/2 cup full-fat whipped cream
- 4 tablespoons Erythritol
- Red food coloring
- 2 cup almond flour
- 4 fresh eggs
- 4 tablespoons butter
- 2 teaspoon baking powder

Directions:
1. Beat the fresh eggs in a bowl and whisk well.
2. Add butter, baking powder, vanilla extract, and whipped cream.
3. Add Erythritol and food coloring.
4. Stir the mixture until well blended and add almond flour.
5. Stir until smooth.

6. Place the mixture in the muffin molds and transfer them to the slow cooker.
7. Cook for 4 hours on High.
8. Cool the cupcakes and serve!

Rhubarb Crumble

Ingredients:

- 1 cup almond flour
- 4 tablespoons butter
- 2 oz walnuts, chopped
- 8 oz rhubarb, chopped
- 1/2 cup Erythritol
- 2 teaspoon vanilla extract

Directions:

1. Mix the vanilla extract, almond flour, and butter.
2. Add walnuts and knead the dough.
3. Chop the dough into small pieces.
4. Cover the bottom of the slow cooker with parchment.
5. Sprinkle it with the small amount of the chopped dough.
6. Add some of the rhubarb and sprinkle it with some Erythritol.

7. Add a layer of the dough again and repeat all the steps until you finish all the ingredients.
8. Cook the crumble for 4 hours on High.
9. Cool the crumble and serve!

Pudding Cake

Ingredients:

- 2 tablespoon cocoa powder
- 4 tablespoons coconut flour
- 4 eggs, beaten
- 4 tablespoons Erythritol
- 2 teaspoon olive oil
- 2 tablespoons butter
- 2 oz dark chocolate
- 2 oz full-fat cream
- 2 teaspoon vanilla extract

Directions:

1. Melt the duck chocolate and combine it with the butter, cream, and vanilla extract.
2. Stir the mixture until smooth.
3. Add the cocoa powder and coconut flour.
4. Add the beaten fresh eggs and Erythritol.
5. Whisk the mixture until smooth.

175

6. Transfer the cake mixture to the slow cooker.
7. Cook for 4 hours on High.
8. Serve the cooked cake after 25 minutes of chilling!

Pineapple Cheese Cake

Ingredients:

- 1/2 cup of sour cream
- 2 tablespoon of vanilla extract
- 2 cups of mixed nuts, crushed
- 2 tablespoons of unsalted butter, melted
- 1/2 cup of raspberries
- 8oz. ricotta cheese
- 2 tablespoon of sugar-free pineapple extract
- 1/2 cup of erythritol
- 2 fresh eggs

Directions:

1. Start by blending the Nuts with butter in the mixer.
2. Spread this Nuts mixture in the greased Crockpot firmly.

3. Now beat the remaining filling Ingredients: except berries in a blender until smooth.
4. Add this cream filling to the Nutty crust and spread evenly.
5. Cover its lid and cook for 6 hours on Low setting.
6. Once done, remove its lid of the crockpot carefully.
7. Allow it to cool and refrigerate for 25 hours.
8. Garnish with berries.
9. Serve.